LOSING BELLY FAT IN NO TIME:

Effective Tips and Healthy Foods That Help Melts Fats.

Martha J. Jones

Table of contents

CHAPTER 1

Belly fat

Belly fat refers to fat around the abdomen. There are two forms of abdominal fat:

- Visceral: This fat surrounds a person's organs.
- Subcutaneous: This is fat that resides beneath the skin.

This form is less detrimental to health and acts as a layer of protection for your organs as well as insulation to regulate body temperature. Health issues from visceral fat are more hazardous than having subcutaneous fat. People may make several lifestyles and nutritional modifications to lose abdominal fat. There are various reasons why individuals accumulate belly fat, including poor nutrition, lack of exercise, and stress. Improving diet, boosting exercise, and making other lifestyle adjustments may all assist.

Why is belly fat dangerous?

Being overweight is one of the biggest causes of serious illnesses.

Excess abdominal fat may raise the risk of:

Heart disease

heart attacks

high blood pressure

stroke

type 2 diabetes

asthma

breast cancer

colon cancer

dementia

Why does belly fat normally form?

Weight growth as a whole is a bit tricky but "belly fat normally arises from ingesting too many calories, which promotes weight gain," explains Keri Gans, R.D.,

That said, you actually can't control where fat accumulates in your body.

"We have absolutely no control on where that weight goes," Gans explains. "It normally ends up on our tummy or hips and thighs according to one's genetics, sex, and/or age."

Food that causes belly fats

1. White Bread

If you're thinking not all bread is nasty, you're correct. It's highly refined, white bread that should be avoided while you're aiming to decrease abdominal fat. Studies have shown that eating healthy grains will lessen visceral fat deposits in your gut, whereas consuming processed grains leads to more.

2. Diet soda.

If you want to get your beach body back, you should take out sugary drinks and replace them with diet ones, right? Sorry, but that's simply wrong. Much research has established a link between the intake of diet drinks and greater waist circumference. What's more, diet soda users had a larger proportion of belly fat than individuals who don't consume the beverage, research in the Journal of the American Geriatrics Society revealed. Why? Researchers suspect diet soda consumers may overestimate how many calories they're "saving," and then overeat.

Instead, sip on some white tea. This brew blocks the formation of new fat cells and helps the body break down stored fat, according to a Nutrition & Metabolism study. That implies that even when you overindulge, it's tougher for your body to retain the extra calories in your body.

3. Fruit Juice.

It's natural, it's filled with Vitamin C—what could go wrong? Well, although 100% fruit juice is a healthier alternative than sugary beverages like Sunny D, even the all-natural kind still carries up to 36 grams of sugar per cup—about the same amount of sugar you would receive if you ate four Krispy Kreme glazed doughnuts. What's more, most of the sweetness in juice comes from fructose, a kind of sugar connected with the formation of visceral adipose tissue—yep, that's belly fat.

Instead, your best bet is to stay with plain ol' H2O. But there is a way to add some taste to those glasses of water. You may add fresh sliced fruit like oranges and grapefruit. The secret, however, is to keep the peels on citrus peels are rich in the antioxidant d-limonene, a potent chemical that helps drain out toxins from the body and enables it to release stored visceral fat.

4. Rib-Eye Steak

Wait—don't chuck your steak knife at us just yet! Studies reveal that eating the appropriate cuts of steak may truly help shrink your midsection. But rib-eye, along with T-bone and New York Strip, is one of the three fattiest cuts. Researchers of one research discovered that having a diet high in fatty, fresh red meat is positively related to abdominal obesity and bigger waist circumference.

5. Chocolate

Let's start by making it clear that not all chocolate is evil. In reality, dark chocolate is swimming in health advantages, and according to research published in Heart, consuming up to 3.5 ounces of chocolate a day may help lessen your risk of heart disease. Plus, it may help decrease abdominal fat! But it's milk chocolate that is the trouble. Milk chocolate bars are filled up with sugar and often containing a ton of calories. An American Journal of Clinical Nutrition research indicated that the food that was connected with the largest weight gain was chocolate bars. Just be careful to stay away from those milk chocolate bars!

6. Canned Soup

Again, when it comes to canned soups you're going to want to want to make sure you're picking the appropriate ones. See, there are lots of soup alternatives that sneak in a ton of salt, which not only creates tummy bloat but also may increase your appetite and hamper your capacity to realize when you're full.

7. Potato Chips

In the race to uncover the worst conceivable meal for your gut, Harvard researchers think they have a winner. It's not simply that potato chips are rich in saturated fat, causing belly fat accumulation. It's not simply that they're coated with salt, producing mid-level bloat. It's not even a pure calorie play—there are lots of more caloric goodies out there. What makes potato chips so epically bad for your belly is not what they have, but what they lack: the ability to make you feel satisfied. A handful of chips can turn into a big empty bag in no time.

8. Frozen Coffee Drinks

Coffee by itself isn't bad for your waistline, but if you're frequently sipping on frozen coffee drinks, then you've just met your problem. Most of the time, these high-calorie drinks are packed with sugar and dairy. Plus, a 2017 study published in Public Health found that nearly 70% of coffee drinkers had their cup of Joe with caloric add-ins including sugar and creamers.

9. Pizza

Even if there are some veggies sprinkled on top, it's important to keep in mind that pizza is still in fact, well, pizza. It's the second biggest contributor of saturated fat to the American diet (just below cheese itself), and most slices serve up half a day's worth of the artery clogger. Researchers have found that, unlike other fats, the saturated variety is the most likely to be stored in the stomach. You'll want to avoid any of the unhealthiest pizzas in America, that's for sure.

10. Low-Fat Pastries

Some people see the label "low fat" and think it's the healthier option. But don't let the tricky terminology fool you. These muffins and treats are typically loaded up with processed flour, tend to be high in sugar, and can be high in sodium, too. These are all components that add up to putting on the belly fat.

11. Pretzels

Pretzels seem like they're a better option than potato chips, and we already know chips are a no-go. Sorry to disappoint, but pretzels are just as bad, as they are loaded up with salt. One study published in the Journal of Nutrition even uncovered how salt confuses the biological processes that tell you when you're full. Essentially, you just end up eating more, which leads to weight gain, and it'll go straight to your belly.

12. Cereal

Not all cereal is bad, but the sugary, colorful kind you most likely ate as a kid? That's the stuff that will lead to excess belly fat. Plenty of cereals are high in sugar, yet low in fiber and protein, so soon enough, you'll feel hungry again. Plus, eating a healthy breakfast every day can help you lose weight more quickly. One study found that 78% of participants who lose 30 pounds or more kept the weight off by eating breakfast daily. As long as you're eating the right kind of breakfast!

13. French Fries

Any fat-laden bad carb-fest will make you gain weight, but there's something almost magical about the effects of fried spuds on your body's fat-storage system. And by magical, we don't mean in a good way. See, one longitudinal Harvard research discovered that persons who ate fries frequently acquired more than three pounds of body weight every four years; throughout the length of the study, the french fry eaters accumulated 13 pounds of belly fat from fries alone!

So what can you have instead? Homemade sweet potato fries that are baked, not fried. A simple switch that will keep that abdominal fat away.

14.Ice Cream

This one is tough to watch, but filling up on ice cream every night isn't going to help you lose that weight—going it's to lead you to pack more on. And why is that? Well, because of all the sugar you consume, ice cream is a carb-heavy meal, and if you happen to eat a lot of refined carbs, this might result in belly fat deposition, So maybe it's better not to eat a pint every night . . .

15. Trans fats

Trans fats are among the unhealthiest fats. While minor quantities of trans fat exist in nature, they're typically manufactured for the food system by adding hydrogen to unsaturated fats in order to make them more stable and enable them to be solid at room temperature. Trans fats are widely utilized in baked goods and packaged meals as a cheap — but effective — alternative for butter, lard, and higher-cost commodities.

Artificial trans fats have been demonstrated to promote inflammation, which may lead to insulin resistance, heart disease, some forms of cancer, and several other disorders. However, ruminant trans fats, which are present naturally in dairy and meat products, do not have the same harmful health consequences.

The American Heart Association advises severely restricting or altogether avoiding artificial trans fats. Many nations, notably the United States and Canada, have outlawed the use of trans fats in food items owing to their detrimental impact on health.

Though it's considered that trans fat may also lead to visceral fat — and has been related to bad health throughout previous decades — there's a little contemporary study on the matter. Even with many nations having taken efforts to restrict or prohibit the use of artificial trans fats in the food supply, it's crucial to still read the nutrition label if you're uncertain.

16.Low fiber diet

Fiber is highly essential for overall health and weight control.

Some forms of fiber may help you feel full, balance hunger hormones, and control your appetite.

In observational research including 1,114 men and women, soluble fiber consumption was related to lower belly fat. For each 10-gram increase in soluble fiber, there was a 3.7% reduction in belly fat formation.

Diets heavy in refined carbohydrates and poor in fiber seem to have the opposite impact on hunger and weight gain, including increases in belly fat.

One big research including 2,854 people indicated that high-fiber whole grains were related to lower abdominal fat, whereas processed grains were connected to increased abdominal fat.

CHAPTER 2

Food That Melts Stubborn Belly Fat

Incorporate these foods into your diet for a smaller midsection.

Looking to melt your middle? Don't worry, it's a lot simpler to accomplish than you think. All you have to do is integrate five distinct food types, each of which helps to battle inflammation, enhance metabolism, and—most important of all—turn off your fat genes and reverse your body's predisposition to accumulate fat. These greatest meals to burn belly fat are intended to give protein, fiber, and healthy fats at every meal to help improve metabolism and battle hunger. They'll increase your amounts of macronutrients to shut down your hereditary

fat-storage systems, while also limiting excess sweets, processed carbs, and additives that are known to upset the stomach and contribute to inflammation and weight gain.
The outcome will be not just rapid, effortless weight reduction but an almost instant sensation of vitality, a smaller midsection, and a lighter body. Read on for the meals that melt stubborn abdominal fat,

1. Eggs

Eggs are the single finest dietary source of the B vitamin choline, which is a vital ingredient involved in the formation of all the body's cell membranes. Two eggs will offer you half your day's amount; only beef liver has more. And believe us, starting your day with a slab of beef liver does not make for a great morning.

But as more and more study is done into the processes of fat genes, the importance of eggs has only risen. Choline shortage is connected directly to the genes that promote visceral fat storage, notably in the liver. One of the reasons heavy drinkers develop fatty liver is that alcohol undercuts the body's ability to process choline. Yet, according to the 2005 National Health and Nutrition Examination Survey, just a tiny minority of all Americans consume daily diets that meet the U.S. Institute of Medicine's Adequate Intake of 425 milligrams for women and 550 milligrams for men. Start your day with eggs, and enjoy some additional sources like lean meat and shellfish

2. Red fruit

More and more studies have started to indicate that certain fruits are better at battling belly fat than others. And the master fruits all have one thing in common; they're red, or at least reddish. These fruits include ruby red grapefruit, tart cherries, raspberries, strawberries, Pink Lady apples, melons, plums, peaches, and nectarines.

3. Olive oil—and other healthful fats

Though it may seem counterintuitive to add fat to a meal if you're trying to lose fat, eating a moderate portion of unsaturated fats, like the kind found in olive oil, avocados, and nuts, can ward off the munchies and keep you full by regulating hunger hormones. A study published in Nutrition Journal found that participants who ate half a fresh avocado with lunch reported a 40% decreased desire to eat for hours afterward. Changing the kind of fat in your diet will also help you increase your intake of omega-3 fatty acids while reducing omega-6 fats (found in vegetable oil and fried foods); upping your ratio of omega-3s to omega-6s has been proven to improve metabolic health and reduce inflammation.

4. Beans, brown rice, oats, and other beneficial fiber

Grains have a poor name because of their carbohydrate content. And now, more and more studies are looking at the impacts of gluten, the protein present in wheat, not only as a culprit in weight gain but because of suspected long-term health repercussions including Alzheimer's and heart disease.

But not all grains are created equal. Gluten-free whole grains like quinoa contain a nutrient called betaine, an amino acid that positively influences the genetic mechanism for insulin resistance and visceral fat.

So stop thinking in terms of "grains" or "carbs" and start thinking about beneficial fiber. The correct fiber sources give your body energy and fuel lean muscle mass while keeping you full all day. In addition to filling fiber, some of the best foods that melt belly fat include beans, lentils, oats, quinoa, and brown rice contain magnesium and chromium—two incredible nutrients that combat cortisol (a stress hormone that directs fat to be stored around the waist) and keep down insulin production (high levels of the hormone also encourage fat to pile on around the belly) (high levels of the hormone also encourage fat to pile on around the belly).

5. Extra plant protein

Plant-based protein powders offer a low-sugar, high-fiber alternative to popular dairy-based supplements. Research from the University of Tampa that compared plant protein to whey showed it to be as efficient in changing body composition and boosting muscle repair and development. But with less sugar and a better lipid profile, plant-based proteins will help boost your intestinal health at the same time as they're nourishing your muscles. Hemp, rice, and pea proteins are all terrific possibilities; however, you'll want to ensure you're receiving a complete protein with a full amino acid profile, which is why a mix that incorporates all three is ideal.

6. Lean meat and fish

Protein is poison to belly fat, and the building block of a lean, toned tummy. When you consume protein, your body needs to waste a lot of calories in digestion—about 25 calories for every 100 calories you eat (compared with just 10 to 15 calories for fats and carbohydrates) (compared with only 10 to 15 calories for fats and carbs). Protein is also more filling. Research published in the American Journal of Clinical Nutrition demonstrated that a meal that's high in protein as opposed to carbohydrates promotes satiety by decreasing the hunger-stimulating hormone ghrelin.

Now, you may be tempted to grab one of those costly protein bars instead of sitting down for a nice dinner. But the result isn't the same. Not only are you receiving a lot of added sugar and chemicals, but you're not getting the same fat-fighting results. Studies reveal that your body spends more calories digesting healthy meals than it does processed items. In addition, lean meats are crucial sources of choline, which we have established is a food that helps turn off the genetic triggers that lead to fatty liver—a new pandemic connected to visceral fat—and methionine and vitamin B12, which unplug genes associated to diabetes and weight gain.

7. Leafy greens, green tea, and brilliantly colored veggies

Low-energy-density foods like vegetables are key for melting belly fat, since they contribute critical nutrients, satisfying fiber, and bulk to meals, all for relatively few calories. Bright hues signify that the veggies are rich in polyphenols, micronutrients that aid to decrease diet-induced inflammation. Green tea has catechins, some of which may "switch off" the genetic triggers for diabetes and obesity. And veggies, particularly the leafy sort, have a low glycemic load—meaning they fill your body full of nutrients without creating a surge in blood sugar. More significantly, eating more green vegetables in a balanced diet may enhance dietary fiber consumption, improve digestive health, and aid in weight control. Plant-based meals that are high in minerals and fiber, such as dark leafy greens, can promote satiety.

8. Your favorite spices and tastes

A new study has discovered that piperine—which is emitted when the waiter from an expensive restaurant uses that enormous pepper grinder in front of your face—has some remarkable magical properties. In animal experiments, piperine has been proven to treat depression, inflammation, and arthritis and increase the activity of other nutrients. In human research, it's been found to boost your capacity to achieve a good tan while spending less time in the sun. Who knew all that could come from a simple pepper grinder?

Research is revealing that herbs, spices, and flavorings do more than provide more bite to your cuisine and help you minimize salt consumption. Yellow mustard seeds have high levels of anti-cancer compounds called glucosinolates; cinnamon has been linked to improved insulin response, and compounds in turmeric and horseradish have been shown to impact the behavior of your fat-storage genes, while ginger packs high levels of health-boosting phytonutrients. Bottom line: adding yellow, black, and brown spices to your meals means you're enhancing the health advantages across the board, while also soothing your urge for additional salt and sugar.

9. Dark chocolate

The advantages of dark chocolate keep stacking up: mental clarity, improved blood pressure, and decreased hunger. A 2014 research discovered that a specific kind of antioxidant in cocoa protected laboratory mice from accumulating extra weight and actually decreased their blood sugar levels. In 2018, Louisiana State University also conducted a study and found that gut microbes in one stomach ferment chocolate and boost our body's production of heart-healthy polyphenolic compounds, including butyrate, a fatty acid that decelerates the behavior of genes linked to insulin resistance and inflammation. Add fruit to the chocolate to promote fermentation and the release of the chemicals! But make sure you're picking the proper type of chocolate: Look for a cacao concentration of 70% or more, and steer clear from Dutch cocoa, since the Dutching process removes up to 77% of the beneficial components in chocolate.

10. SPICY CHILI PEPPERS

Bring on the heat! Spicy chili peppers contain capsaicin, a chemical known to induce satiety and reduce calorie intake, "It also helps stimulate fat burning. Enjoy capsaicin by sprinkling ground cayenne or chili pepper over food or in drinks such as tea or lemon water, or cook spicy peppers into stews, chilis, and soups." Or, you know, pop raw ones straight, If you're courageous!

11. SEA VEGETABLES

They may not be entirely popular but there's ample reason to add marine jewels like nori, hijiki, wakame, arame, and kombu into your normal diet. With omega-3 fatty acids not found in other plant meals, sea veggies (or seaweed) are inflammation-fighting powerhouses, "Omega-3 fatty acids are effective inflammation-fighters, so sea veggies may boost your body's capacity to regulate inflammation and may contribute to a flatter tummy." Note: Store-bought seaweed snacks may carry a lot of salt (which can lead to bloat), so be careful to review nutrition labels before purchase.

12.BROCCOLI

"A research published in the Journal of the Academy of Nutrition and Dietetics indicated that dark green vegetables, including broccoli, may help decrease abdominal fat, "The research also revealed that these vegetables may potentially lessen risk factors for type 2 diabetes."

13.BEANS

"Beans are the ultimate weight reduction food,"They have the ideal macronutrient composition (a perfect ratio of fiber and protein) to ensure satiety with few calories and they also happen to be versatile, cheap, and user-friendly. You should eat at least one and a half cups of beans a day to support weight loss without feeling hungry."

Beans are also abundant in both plant-based protein and carbohydrates which promotes satiety and metabolism making them a wonderful and economical alternative to help get rid of abdominal fat.

14.NUTS

"Nuts are unexpectedly a fantastic diet to promote weight reduction. Although they're high in calories, they've been related to weight reduction and weight loss maintenance," adds Hever. "Researchers say this is owing to the fact that nuts enhance fullness, hence leading to compensation of calories elsewhere in the diet. Also, nuts have been demonstrated to enhance resting metabolism." A higher metabolism may help wash away any bloating, so this is certainly a positive for getting into your thin pants or favorite evening dress.

15. Walnuts

Walnuts are high in monounsaturated fats – they're an excellent heart-healthy snack compared with other grab-and-go products like chips or pretzels. One ounce comes in at under 200 calories and includes 4 grams of protein and 2 grams of fiber. But you'll discover that this nut happens to be incredibly satiating. The previous study has demonstrated that walnuts, in particular, assist in suppressing cravings that you may have had in between meals in the past. Walnuts also give nearly double the number of antioxidant polyphenols than many other nuts like peanuts and tree nuts as revealed by first research. Research results demonstrate that as compared to control meals, walnut-enriched diets resulted in much larger reductions in total and LDL cholesterol and triglyceride levels. They also include prebiotics, an indigestible fiber that feeds probiotics that have been demonstrated to favorably benefit gut flora. Enjoy walnuts on their own or add them to grain meals like quinoa, wheat berries, or couscous. Chopped walnuts may be integrated into ground meat meals, and they are fantastic to use for extra texture and crunch in baked products.

16.MILK

"A research published in a study published in Nutrition Journal connected calcium and vitamin D supplementation over 12 weeks with belly fat reduction in obese and overweight college students," adds Amidor. "These individuals also cut their calories over this period. Although the research was done using supplements, milk is rich in both calcium and vitamin D, and may be part of a healthy weight reduction regimen.

17.Yogurt

In the same line as milk, dairy products such as plain or Greek yogurt are also among the greatest foods for belly fat removal. According to a 2014 research, high-protein snacks such as yogurts perform wonderfully as the best approach to reduce belly fat as they help manage your appetite, counter hunger, and lower your total food consumption.

18.FARRO

Everybody loves their quinoa, but it's time to elevate this less-popular grain to superfood status.

If you are bored of eating quinoa and brown rice all the time, farro is another fantastic wholegrain choice. It is abundant in fiber and protein; hence, ingesting it is another effective approach to decreasing abdominal fat. While processed carbohydrates and sugar are the major culprits for increasing belly obesity, whole grains are in another category entirely, "Intact grains [i.e., ones that haven't been stripped of their nutrients, as is usually the case with 'white' choices] include fiber which delays digestion and absorption of the grains, which in turn decreases the amount of insulin generated by the body." What does this imply for you? The less insulin your body produces means less abdominal fat attaching itself to your belly.

19.GARLIC

It seems odd to feed the microbiome items with antimicrobial characteristics, but studies demonstrate that garlic only goes after harmful, inflammation-causing bacteria while leaving beneficial bacteria intact. It's also high in inulin, the fiber that helps the body digest meals more effectively and steadies blood sugar. Add fresh chopped garlic to tomato-mozzarella salads and stir-fries, or sprinkle garlic powder over meats and fish before grilling.

20.OATMEAL

Having a substantial cup of oatmeal for breakfast isn't only tasty, it's healthy for your waistline. " The whole grains not only absorb water to make you feel more full, but they're also high in soluble fiber to keep you feeling satisfied for long periods.

However, oats are not just excellent weight-loss foods. They are fantastic for your overall health as they lower your blood cholesterol levels, boost the immune system, and regulate your blood glucose levels. Have some oats as your breakfast, make some oat pancakes, or add some oat flour to your smoothies to make them more nutritious and filling.

However, Don't just restrict oats to breakfast; they can be turned into oat flour for baking and even converted into delicious oat bowls for lunch or dinnertime. Does your smoothie leave you starving after an hour? Try adding in a scoop of nutrient-dense oats. They blend well and add a good source of dietary fiber to your smoothie to keep you fuller for longer.

21.GRAPEFRUIT

If you have a big-time sweet craving, grabbing a grapefruit might help cut down on calories from late-night snacks. "The great thing about grapefruit, and citrus fruits in general, is that they deliver a powerful, fulfilling taste that seldom gets chanced by sweets," Taub-Dix explains. "A grapefruit or citrus fruit after dinner might discourage you from reaching for a sugary dessert." Yeah, that's right: a 52-calorie grapefruit may satisfy just as much as a 400-calorie piece of chocolate cake. Sorry, brain, but you just got played.

22.CHIA SEEDS

They are filled with key nutrients like omega-3s, fiber, and proteins, all of which help speed up your metabolic rate and take longer to digest, keeping you content for longer and minimizing excessive snacking.

Chia seeds can appear little, but they are formidable. The small seeds may swell 10 times their weight in water, turning into a gel-like material (chia pudding, anyone?) that can keep you satisfied for extended periods, helping you take in fewer calories overall and lose weight around your waist.

23. SPIRULINA

If you're not ready to ingest full-on seaweed pieces just yet (you're not alone!), try spirulina. Adding a spoonful of the lovely blue-green algae into your smoothie every day can help control cravings, prevent disease, and — of course — help you burn off unsightly belly fat.

24. Chickpeas

Whether you are a vegan, vegetarian, or meat lover, if you are wanting to get rid of belly fat, chickpeas should be on your shopping list. They are an excellent source of plant-based protein and fiber, two components that perform well for both fat reduction and weight loss.

25.Salmon

This popular protein is fairly low in calories (under 200 calories for a 3-ounce serving) and makes an ideal meal choice because it's packed with polyunsaturated fatty acids called omega-3 fatty acids. Omega-3s are essential as the body can't produce them; we must get them regularly from our diet. These nutritious fatty acids can contribute to a healthy heart as well as benefit cholesterol, triglycerides, inflammation, and even blood clotting. Plus, the combo of healthy fats and protein in salmon makes it very satisfying. Like eggs, which are rich in omega-3 fatty acids which work great for fat burning. It is also rich in lean protein which enhances satiety and your metabolism.

26.Peanut Butter And Other Nut Butters

Instead of spreading sugary-filled jams and jellies on bread, switch to peanut butter (or other nut jars of butter instead). You can also have peanut butter as a snack with fruits and vegetables like apples or celery. One serving of natural peanut butter can have up to 8 grams of protein and up to 4 grams of fiber per serving which keeps you satiated for longer and boosts your metabolism.

27.Pumpkin

Pumpkin makes it onto this list of the 32 foods that burn belly fat fast due to its high amounts of fiber and low calories. Not only will it keep you satiated for longer preventing unhealthy snacking, but it doesn't threaten your daily energy requirement.

28.Sunflower Seeds

They are packed with polyunsaturated fats which are good for your heart health and decrease the risk of type II diabetes. Sunflower seeds are among the foods that burn belly fat fast because they are also filled with protein and fiber.

29.Quinoa

Not only is it rich in fiber, but it also provides all nine necessary amino acids which make it one of the finest meals for weight reduction. One 2017 study revealed that this grain helped lower triglyceride levels in overweight and obese subjects as well as helping them lose weight and waist circumference.

Quinoa provides a filling and nutrient-rich alternative to refined carbohydrates like white pasta and white rice. Bonus: It doesn't disrupt blood sugar levels due to its low glycemic index. All in all, quinoa is a must-add to any kitchen to promote sustained weight management.

Considered a seed, quinoa is available in several varieties including red, black, and white. It has a delicious nutty taste and is fantastic as a side dish, swapped for rice in stuffed peppers, and even included in breakfast bowls as a replacement for oats. If you haven't tried quinoa before, try it as a side dish for a weeknight dinner.

30. Peas

Whether you choose to have green peas or split peas, both options are great weight loss foods as they are high in vitamins, minerals, and fiber. They also contain complex carbohydrates, which are a good source of energy. Peas are also high in protein which keeps you fuller for longer and boosts your metabolism.

31.Blueberries

According to studies done on mice, a diet rich in blueberries can contribute to losing abdominal fat. The mice in the research exhibited a decrease in their belly fat, triglycerides, and overall body weight .Blueberries are also incredibly abundant in vitamins that improve your immune system.

32.Apples

Whether you cut it up in a salad, eat it whole, or add it to a morning smoothie, consuming apples is one option to get rid of belly fat. According to a 2012 study, apples contain ursolic acid, a compound that increases brown fat (the good fat), and muscle mass (which boosts metabolism), and helps decrease diet-induced obesity.

33. Tea

Whether you are consuming green tea, black tea, or oolong tea, this drink makes it on this list of the best 32 foods that burn belly fat fast due to the presence of catechins. Catechins have long been praised for their potential fat and weight loss benefits.

In one 2012 study, the group that consumed catechins in green tea lost 0.6 kgs, 1.7 kgs, and

2.3 kgs of lean mass, weight, and body fat mass, respectively. Consuming a beverage containing green tea catechins (625mg/d) may enhance exercise-induced loss of abdominal fat and improve triglyceride levels.

34.Kiwi Fruit

This fruit rounds up our list of 32 foods that burn belly fat fast as it is a great source of plant-based fiber and prebiotics that feeds the friendly bacteria that help your metabolism function optimally.

35.Fermented Foods

Fermented foods such as kefir, sauerkraut, kombucha, fermented or raw cheeses, raw apple cider vinegar, kimchi (fermented cabbage), natto, miso, or tempeh are great for weight and belly fat loss. This is because they contain probiotics (good bacteria like Lactobacillus and Bifidobacterium) which have been shown to aid this process.

36.Lentils

Plant-based proteins like lentils might prove to be an effective weight reduction meal since they are also rich in fiber. These small protein-filled pieces of plant-based deliciousness are a fantastic complement to soups or salads since they make a meal seem so much more substantial. The fiber and resistant starch inside lentils might help you eat fewer calories between meals. Resistant starch is a form of carbohydrate that resists digestion in the small intestine, instead fermenting in the large intestine and functioning as a prebiotic to feed the beneficial bacteria in the gut while the fiber ferments.

At roughly 120 calories per half cup and an astonishing 8 grams of fiber, lentils are one of the high-fiber foods that are ideal for weight reduction and an overall healthy diet. Research on pulses like lentils, chickpeas, dried peas, and others shows that they may aid in mild weight reduction even without deliberate calorie limitation. Lentils are extremely low in salt and saturated fat, making them a heart-healthy option too.

Lentils come in a range of distinct hues and offer depth and earthiness to any dish. Toss them in chopped salads or grain bowls, and add them to meat mixes like chilis and stews to provide extra bulk and nutrition. You can even use a food processor to crush down lentils into a paste to make a vegetable burger or vegan meatballs.

37. Asparagus

This tasty vegetable is a weight-loss-friendly option since it's low in calories, rich in water content, and includes fiber too. One medium spear of asparagus is just 3 calories and has fantastic texture and crunch. This cholesterol-free, fat-free, and low-sodium choice provides a delightful accent to numerous recipes. What's crucial with asparagus — and any vegetable — is the preparation: Try air frying it for a great crispy texture without the added need for heavy fats. As a prebiotic-filled plant, asparagus jacks up the benefits of soups, kinds of pasta, and omelets, and makes an easy and delightful side dish. Also, try combining asparagus stalks with other crudité and dipping them in hummus.

38.Almonds

Almonds keep your stomach full for a long time thanks to their healthy fat and protein composition. They are fantastic sources of nutrients for vegetarians to burn fat. They are also rich in omega-3 fatty acids that improve energy and metabolism.

CHAPTER 3

Effective Tips to Lose Belly Fat

1. Follow a Calorie Deficit

Watching how much you eat as well as how many calories you burn each day is frequently the first port of call we handle. But instead of starving ourselves, the idea is to follow something known as a 'calorie deficit."This means you are ingesting less food than what your body is burning during the day.

Many factors may help you lose weight and belly fat, but ingesting fewer calories than your body requires for weight maintenance is crucial. Keeping a food journal or utilizing an online meal tracker or app may help you manage your calorie consumption. This technique has been proven to be useful for weight reduction.

In addition, food-tracking programs assist you to examine your consumption of protein, carbohydrates, fiber, and micronutrients. Many also allow you to record your exercise and physical activity.

As a general weight-loss suggestion, it's always a good idea to keep track of what you're eating. Keeping a food diary or utilizing an online meal tracker are two of the most common methods to achieve this.

2. Eat lots of soluble fiber.

Soluble fiber absorbs water and produces a gel that helps slow down food as it goes through your digestive system. Studies suggest that this kind of fiber improves weight reduction by making you feel full, so you naturally eat less. It may also lower the number of calories your body absorbs from meals.

What's more, soluble fiber may help combat belly fat. Make an effort to eat high-fiber meals every day.

Excellent sources of soluble fiber include:

flax seeds

shirataki noodles

Brussels sprouts

avocados

legumes

blackberries.

Beans, peas, and lentils

Nuts and Seeds

Berries

Squash

Broccoli

Whole Grains

Soluble fiber may help you to lose weight by increasing fullness and reducing calorie absorption. Try to include plenty of high-fiber foods in your weight loss diet.

3. Avoid foods that contain trans fats(focus on healthy fats)

Science has ruled that all fats aren't created equal. Many of us know that the fat in an avocado is healthier than that of fat found in fast food. One research went further and revealed that individuals who ate avocados tended to have less abdominal fat than those who don't. And part of this was due to their monounsaturated fat called oleic acid which is also present in olive oil.

Trans fats are created by pumping hydrogen into unsaturated fats, such as soybean oil. They're found in some kinds of margarine and spreads and are also often added to packaged foods, but many food producers have stopped using them. These fats have been linked to inflammation, heart disease, insulin resistance, and abdominal fat gain. To help reduce belly fat and protect your health, read ingredient labels carefully and stay away from products that contain trans fats. These are commonly classified as partly hydrogenated fats.

Some studies have connected a high diet of trans fat to higher belly fat growth. Regardless of whether you're wanting to lose weight, limiting your intake of trans fat is a good idea.

4. Don't drink too much alcohol.

Alcohol may offer health benefits in small amounts, but it's critically harmful if you drink too much. Research suggests that too much alcohol may also lead you to gain belly fat. Excessive alcohol use has been connected with increased belly fat. If you need to trim your waistline, consider drinking alcohol in moderation or quitting entirely.

5. Eat a high-protein diet.

Protein is an extremely important nutrient for weight management. High protein intake increases the release of the fullness hormone PYY, which decreases appetite and promotes fullness. Protein also raises your metabolic rate and helps you to retain muscle mass during weight loss. Many observational studies show that people who eat more protein tend to have less abdominal fat than those who eat a lower protein diet.

Be careful to consume a nutritious protein source at every meal, such as:

meat

fish

eggs

dairy

whey protein

beans

High protein meals, such as fish, lean meat, and beans, are great if you're seeking to shed any additional pounds around your waist.

6. Reduce your stress levels

Stress may help you gain belly fat by stimulating the adrenal glands to release cortisol, which is also known as the stress hormone.

Research shows that high cortisol levels increase appetite and drive abdominal fat storage,

What's more, women who already have a large waist tend to produce more cortisol in response to stress. Increased cortisol further adds to fat gain around the middle.

It's something we all experience from time to time. But sadly stress and particularly stress-eating has a huge impact on our waistlines.

"Without realizing, stress can make you gain belly fat by triggering cortisol hormones," explains Rob. "When your cortisol levels are running high your appetite will increase, meaning you will not only put on more weight, but it will also be harder to lose weight."

To help reduce belly fat, engage in pleasurable activities that relieve stress. Practicing yoga or meditation can be effective methods.

Stress may encourage fat growth around your waist. Minimizing stress should be one of your priorities if you're trying to lose weight.

7. Avoid sugary food

Sugar includes fructose, which has been related to various chronic illnesses when taken in excess. These include heart disease, type 2 diabetes, obesity, and fatty liver disease.

Observational studies demonstrate an association between excessive sugar consumption and increased belly fat.

It's crucial to recognize that more than simply refined sugar may contribute to abdominal fat growth. Even healthy sweets, such as genuine honey, should be used sparingly. Excessive sugar consumption is a key cause of weight gain in many individuals. Limit your consumption of confectionery and processed meals rich in added sugar.

8. Cut down on carbohydrates — particularly refined carbs

Reducing your carb consumption may be quite useful for shedding weight, even abdominal fat. Diets with under 50 grams of carbohydrates per day induce belly fat reduction in those who are overweight, those at risk for type 2 diabetes, and women with the polycystic ovarian syndrome (PCOS).

You don’t have to follow a rigorous low-carb diet. Some studies show that merely replacing 6) refined carbohydrates with unprocessed starchy carbs may improve metabolic health and minimize abdominal obesity.

A high diet of refined carbohydrates is related to increased abdominal fat. Consider lowering your carb consumption or substituting refined carbohydrates in your diet with healthy carb sources, such as whole grains, legumes, or vegetables.

9. Avoid sugar-sweetened drinks

You don't have to be a scientist to realize that ingesting high amounts of sugar may lead to an inflow of pounds.

Sugar-sweetened beverages are loaded with liquid fructose, which can make you gain belly fat.

Studies show that sugary drinks lead to increased fat in the liver. One 10-week study found significant abdominal fat gain in people who consumed high fructose beverages.

Sugary beverages appear to be even worse than high-sugar foods.

Since your brain doesn't process liquid calories the same way it does solid ones, you're likely to end up consuming too many calories later on and storing them as fat.

To lose belly fat, it's best to completely avoid sugar-sweetened beverages such as:

soda

punch

sweet tea

alcoholic mixers containing sugar

Avoiding all liquid forms of sugar, such as sugar-sweetened drinks, is particularly crucial if you're attempting to drop some excess pounds.

9. Get plenty of restful sleep

Sleep is important for many aspects of your health, including weight. Studies show that people who don't get enough sleep tend to gain more weight, which may include belly fat. A lack of decent sleep, particularly deep sleep, has been scientifically shown to lead to weight gain. A 16-year study involving more than 68,000 women found that those who slept less than 5 hours per night were significantly more likely to gain weight than those who slept 7 hours or more per night.

The condition known as sleep apnea, where breathing stops intermittently during the night, has also been linked to excess visceral fat.

In addition to sleeping at least 7 hours per night, make sure you're getting sufficient quality sleep.

If you suspect you may have sleep apnea or another sleep disorder, speak to a doctor and get treated.

Sleep deprivation is linked to an increased risk of weight gain. Getting enough high-quality sleep should be one of your main priorities if you plan to lose weight and improve your health.

10.Eat fatty fish every week

Fatty fish are incredibly healthy.

They're rich in high-quality protein and omega-3 fats that protect you from disease. Some evidence suggests that these omega-3 fats may also help reduce visceral fat.

Studies in adults and children with fatty liver disease show that fish oil supplements can significantly reduce liver and abdominal fat.

Aim to get 2–3 servings of fatty fish per week. Good choices include:

salmon

herring

sardines

mackerel

anchovies

Eating fatty fish or taking omega-3 supplements may boost your general health. Some data also show it may decrease abdominal fat in persons with fatty liver disease.

11. Avoid sugary food

Sugar includes fructose, which has been related to various chronic illnesses when taken in excess. These include heart disease, type 2 diabetes, obesity, and fatty liver disease. Observational studies demonstrate an association between excessive sugar consumption and increased belly fat.

It's crucial to recognize that more than simply refined sugar may contribute to abdominal fat growth. Even healthy sweets, such as genuine honey, should be used sparingly. Excessive sugar consumption is a key cause of weight gain in many individuals. Limit your consumption of confectionery and processed meals rich in added sugar.

12. Cut down on carbohydrates — particularly refined carbs

Reducing your carb consumption may be quite useful for shedding weight, even abdominal fat. Diets with under 50 grams of carbohydrates per day induce belly fat reduction in those who are overweight, those at risk for type 2 diabetes, and women with the polycystic ovarian syndrome (PCOS).

You don't have to follow a rigorous low-carb diet. Some studies show that merely replacing 6) refined carbohydrates with unprocessed starchy carbs may improve metabolic health and minimize abdominal obesity.

A high diet of refined carbohydrates is related to increased abdominal fat. Consider lowering your carb consumption or substituting refined carbohydrates in your diet with healthy carb sources, such as whole grains, legumes, or vegetables.

13.Avoid sugar-sweetened drinks

You don't have to be a scientist to realize that ingesting high amounts of sugar may lead to an inflow of pounds.

Sugar-sweetened beverages are loaded with liquid fructose, which can make you gain belly fat.

Studies show that sugary drinks lead to increased fat in the liver. One 10-week study found significant abdominal fat gain in people who consumed high fructose beverages.

Sugary beverages appear to be even worse than high-sugar foods.

Since your brain doesn’t process liquid calories the same way it does solid ones, you’re likely to end up consuming too many calories later on and storing them as fat.

To lose belly fat, it's best to completely avoid sugar-sweetened beverages such as:

soda

punch

sweet tea

Stop drinking fruit juice

Although fruit juice delivers vitamins and minerals, it's equally as heavy in sugar as soda and other sweetened drinks.

Drinking high quantities may bring the same danger for belly fat accumulation.

An 8-ounce (240-mL) portion of unsweetened apple juice has 24 grams of sugar, half of which is fructose (58). (58). To help decrease extra belly fat, substitute fruit juice with water, unsweetened iced tea, or sparkling water with a slice of lemon or lime.

When it comes to fat growth, fruit juice may be just as dangerous as a fizzy drink. Consider eliminating all forms of liquid sugar to enhance your probability of effectively reducing weight.

14. Add apple cider vinegar to your diet

Drinking apple cider vinegar offers amazing health advantages, including reducing blood sugar levels.

It includes acetic acid, which has been demonstrated to diminish belly fat accumulation in various animal experiments.

In a 12-week controlled research in males diagnosed with obesity, those who took 1 tablespoon (15 mL) of apple cider vinegar each day dropped half an inch (1.4 cm) off their waists.

1–2 teaspoons (15–30 mL) of apple cider vinegar per day is safe for most individuals and may contribute to minor fat reduction.

However, be careful to dilute it with water, since undiluted vinegar may damage the enamel on your teeth.

If you want to try apple cider vinegar, there's a wide range to pick from online.

Apple cider vinegar may assist you to shed some weight. Animal studies suggest it may help to reduce belly fat.

15.. Eat probiotic foods or take a probiotic supplement

Probiotics are microorganisms present in various meals and supplements. They offer several health advantages, including aiding improve gastrointestinal health and increasing immunological function.

Researchers have shown that various kinds of bacteria play a role in weight management and that having the appropriate balance may aid with weight reduction, especially the loss of belly fat. Those shown to reduce belly fat include members of the Lactobacillus family, such as Lactobacillus fermentum, Lactobacillus amylovorus, and especially Lactobacillus gasseri.

Boosting your body's beneficial bacteria with probiotics is scientifically proven to reduce belly fat.\s"Probiotics are good bacteria which help to restore the balance in your gut, helping to ease and eliminate inflammation that could be the cause of bloating(opens in new tab) or result in difficulties losing weight and shedding fat," nutritionist Rob tells us.

You can find probiotics in healthy yogurts, including some good-for-you greek yogurt.

Probiotic supplements typically contain several types of bacteria, so make sure you purchase one that provides one or more of these bacterial strains.

Taking probiotic supplements may help promote a healthy digestive system. Studies also suggest that beneficial gut bacteria may help promote weight loss.

17. Intermittent fasting

Intermittent fasting has recently become very popular as a weight loss method.

Intermittent fasting is an eating habit that alternates between periods of eating and fasting.

Studies suggest that it may be one of the most effective ways to lose weight and belly fat.

It's an eating pattern that cycles between periods of eating and periods of fasting.

One popular method involves 24-hour fasts once or twice a week. Another consists of fasting every day for 16 hours and consuming all your meals within an 8-hour period.

In a review of trials on intermittent fasting and alternate-day fasting, patients exhibited a 4–7% reduction in belly fat between 6–24 weeks (70). (70).

There's some evidence that intermittent fasting, and fasting in general, may not be as helpful for women as for males. Although certain modified intermittent fasting methods appear to be better options, stop fasting immediately if you experience any negative effects.

18. Drink green tea

Green tea is an exceptionally healthy beverage. It contains caffeine and the antioxidant epigallocatechin gallate (EGCG), both of which appear to boost metabolism.

EGCG is a catechin, which several studies suggest may help you lose belly fat. The effect may be strengthened when green tea consumption is combined with exercise.

Regularly drinking green tea has been linked to weight loss, though it's probably not as effective on its own and best combined with exercise.

19. Drink a lot of water

Hydration is essential for your health overall. And drinking plenty of water(opens in new tab) is especially effective when it comes to weight loss You should strive to drink roughly six to eight glasses of water each day to notice effects," he tells us. "Water helps reduce your hunger and enhances workout performance meaning you burn more." Scientific studies also suggest that water is excellent when seeking to decrease abdominal fat.

One research found that people who drank water before a meal lost 44% more weight than those who didn't. And that this may have accelerated weight reduction by 2kg over 12 weeks.

20. Walk more: Do aerobic exercise (cardio)

Aerobic exercise (cardio) is an effective way to improve your health and burn calories.

Studies also show that it’s one of the most effective forms of exercise for reducing belly fat.

However, results are mixed as to whether

moderate or high-intensity exercise is more beneficial. In any case, the frequency and duration of your exercise program are more important than its intensity.

One study found that postmenopausal women lost more fat from all areas when they did aerobic exercise for 300 minutes per week, compared with those who exercised 150 minutes per week.

Aerobic exercise is an effective weight loss method. Studies suggest it's particularly effective at slimming your waistline.

As David Wiener simply states: "Walking is a form of cardio and cardio burns calories. "

Those wanting to shift some belly fat should try and stretch their legs as often as possible.

Especially as science has highlighted walking as a proven way to lose weight. Research showed that overweight women who walked for 50-70 minutes, 3 days a week, successfully lost more belly fat than those who were sedentary.

Your walking rate also determines how much weight you can lose too. Another study by the British Journal of Sports Medicine showed that those who walked at a pace of 4.6 mph, burned over 50% more calories than those who walked at 3.6 mph and 4.1 mph.

A simple way to up your steps can be as simple as swapping the lift for the stairs on your morning commute. "Most people would believe that going up a few flights of stairs wouldn’t make a difference or it’s a waste of time, but that’s not the case," David Weiner says.

"Keeping your body moving, no matter how will have a tremendous influence on your weight reduction journey and overall wellness."

21. Start Your Day Early

Don't allow additional hours lying in bed to stand between you and a flatter stomach. While getting adequate sleep might assist raise your metabolic rate, sleeping in may negate whatever advantage you'd receive from catching a few more winks. One Obesity research showed that late sleepers who snoozed until 10:45 in the morning ate roughly 250 more calories over the rest of the day while consuming half as many fruits and vegetables as their early bird counterparts. Even worse, they chowed down on more salty, sugary, and trans-fat-laden fast food than those who got up earlier. If you chance to get out of the house early, you're in for an extra metabolic boost; researchers at Northwestern University have shown that persons exposed to only a brief time of early morning sunshine had lower BMIs than their late-waking peers.

22. Eat More Berries Loaded With Antioxidants.

Instead of indulging your sweet desire with refined sugar, switch to berries and have a thinner waistline in no time without exercise. Berries are filled with antioxidants, which may help lower inflammation throughout the body, and a study from the University of Michigan finds that rats fed a cherry-rich diet shaved off a large amount of their belly fat when compared to a control group. Berries like strawberries, raspberries, blueberries, and blackberries are also laden in resveratrol, an antioxidant pigment that has been linked to decreases in belly fat and a lower risk of dementia, to boot.

23. Switch to Sprouted Bread.

While it's often assumed that bread is off-limits when you're trying to lose belly fat, the right bread may actually expedite the process. Switching to sprouted bread can help carb-lovers eager to get their fix without going up a belt size, thanks to the inulin content of sprouted grains. The findings of research published in Nutrition & Metabolism indicate that pre-diabetic study volunteers whose meals were supplemented with inulin shaved off more abdominal fat and overall weight than those whose meal plans didn't carry this nutritious prebiotic fiber.

24. Lift Weights

Do you even lift? If you're serious about getting rid of that belly fat quickly, resistance exercise could well be the secret. Research from the Harvard School of Public Health revealed that adding weight training to adult male test participants' exercises dramatically lowered their risk of abdominal obesity during a multi-year study period, but performing the same amount of cardio had no such benefit. Research from the University of Maryland even revealed that only 16 weeks of weight training raised study participants' metabolic rates by a staggering 7.7 percent, making it simpler to drop those extra inches around your belly.

25. Swap Ketchup for Salsa

Sure, ketchup is yummy, but it's also a significant saboteur when it comes to your weight reduction attempts. Ketchup is laden with sugar — up to four grams per tablespoon — and has little nutritional similarity to the fruit from which it's derived. Luckily, swapping out your ketchup for salsa can help you shave off that belly fat at home without a diet. Fresh tomatoes, like those used in salsa, are loaded with lycopene, which a study conducted at China Medical University in Taiwan links to reductions in both overall fat and waist circumference. If you like your salsa spicy, all the better; the capsaicin in hot peppers, like jalapeños and chipotles, can boost your metabolism, too.

26. Get More Vitamin D

While few would suggest you start hitting up the tanning beds for better health, getting some natural sunlight can help you get rid of belly fat in a matter of weeks. Researchers at the Fred Hutchinson Cancer Research Center showed that vitamin D-deficient overweight women between 50 and 75 who boosted their consumption of the so-called sunshine vitamin dropped more weight and body fat than those who didn't. To practice safe sun, make sure you're limiting yourself to 15 sunscreen-free minutes per day.

27. Set Targets

If you're looking to lose belly fat, it's important to know where you've come from and where you want to get to, so there's nothing wrong with setting yourself a target, even if it's ambitious. In fact, a study published in the Journal of Human Nutrition and Dietetics found setting targets increased the likelihood of achieving "clinically significant weight loss" and, for some, setting 'unrealistic' targets improved their results.

28. Change your lifestyle and combine different methods

Just doing one of the items on this list won't have a big effect on its own. If you want good results, you need to combine different methods that have been shown to be effective.

Interestingly, many of these methods are things generally associated with healthy eating and an overall healthy lifestyle. Therefore, changing your lifestyle for the long term is the key to losing your belly fat and keeping it off.

When you have healthy habits and eat real food, fat loss tends to follow as a natural side effect.

Losing weight and keeping it off is difficult unless you permanently change your dietary habits and lifestyle.

There are no magic solutions to losing belly fat. Weight loss always requires some effort, commitment, and perseverance on your behalf